WHAT IS THE SOUND OF ONE POUND DROPPING?

How to Solve the Riddle of Losing Weight

PATRICIA BRAWLEY PhD, LPC

EXPRESSO
Executive Center 777, Dunsmuir Street Vancouver, BC V71K4
1-888-721-0662 ext 101
info@expressopublishing.com

CONTENTS

CHAPTER 1

GETTING STARTED

"Suffering usually relates to wanting things to be different from the way they are."

—Allan Lokos,
Pocket Peace: Effective Practices for Enlightened Living

I am not different from you. I've been thin, overweight, tired, embarrassed, motivated, and hopeless. Those experiences and many years of study have changed my life and health. I want you to reap the benefits of what I've learned. This is a guide to solve your own riddle about weight and health. You are who matters.

By now you've bought many diet program, consumed hundreds of diet foods and drinks, spent tons of money, and are still going up and down with both your weight and mood. You have a riddle to solve. And I have solutions for you.

Each chapter in this book is short by design. Take in small amounts of information and "chew" on them and reflect on the insights you learn. Give yourself time. There is no rush, but I'm sure you want it NOW. Action steps support this process. Solving the riddle of your weight is the goal of this book.

You do not have to be Buddhist to understand the concept of "koan." A koan is a practice to solve a riddle. A well-used koan is "What is the sound of one hand clapping?" Pondering the answer will leave your mind open or give you an intuitive hit.

The chapters in this book are steps toward solving your koan of "What Is the Sound of One Pound Dropping." The chapters can be used as a guide. You can work through them in any order and at your own pace.

I suggest you write down the action steps in a journal. Your answers will be different from the ones you think in your mind.

Action Step:

What is the riddle of your weight/health you would like to solve? Write down what you know and don't know. For example: I know if I eat Chinese food, I gain two pounds overnight. I don't know why this bothers me if I continue to do it.

What sound do you make when you gain weight?

What does that sound mean to you?

What sound do you make when you lose weight?

What does that sound mean to you?

Whatever you want to change, consider that the reason you got to where you are is your own thinking, and unless you change your subconscious mind, it will be difficult to do it differently over the long haul. You can exercise, work harder, etc., but you get tired and then the pounds come back, the money trickles out of your account and—well, here we are again.

You have to raise the bar. And adopt a corrected course of action. Are you ready? Really. Are you ready? Why or why not?

❦ Action Plan ❦

CHAPTER 2

WHAT IS THE SOUND OF ONE POUND DROPPING?

This is a koan, a riddle. Koans are often brief paradoxical statements or questions used as a practice in Zen Buddhism. The effort to solve a koan/riddle is designed to exhaust the analytic intellect and the will, leaving the mind open for a response on an intuitive level. There are endless numbers of koans but one well-known example: "What is the sound of one hand clapping?"

Do you feel joy if you lose a pound? What does joy sound like to you? Does it sound like laughter? Is the answer "My jeans fit again!" What is your reaction when you step on the scale and see a lower number?

What is the sound you make when you gain a pound? What does that feel like?

Can you see that whether you gain or lose pounds, your mind and feelings are focused on it and you lose sight of the present moment? In other words, you don't know if the birds are singing or not.

We both know that being a certain size does not equal happiness. I'm not promising that. What I am promising is a journey to really understand your body and how your choices, feelings, and health play a role in what you experience as "my body, my weight."

Action Step:

Draw a picture of your family—stick figures allowed. Put yourself in the picture if you left yourself out.

Who did you draw first? Who did you leave out? Notice the proportions of the family members. Do you look like everyone else or one person more than the other? It doesn't matter. We all inherit genes, and we are not doomed because of that fact.

Action Step:

On a different page, draw a representational outline of your body. Write in all the roles you play to others, such as daughter, mother, wife, son, mother-in-law, employee, neighbor, etc. One by one write down characteristics of yourself in each role. Are you friendly to your neighbor, hostile to your boss?

You will eventually notice that "you" are not fixed and rigid and that you move in and out of roles and attitudes. Take one role that you play, such as "friend," and look at your weight problem with the attitude you show to your friends. Identify the roles where you nurture (children, parents, pets). Don't overlook the roles where you harbor negative attitudes and feelings. Which do you feel toward yourself?

Today, assume the role of a person worthy of respect, love, and one who has the ability to solve problems. Extend a nurturing attitude toward yourself.

> "The most fundamental aggression to ourselves, the most fundamental harm we can do to ourselves, is to remain ignorant by not having the courage and the respect to look at ourselves honestly and gently." — Pema Chödrön, *When Things Fall Apart: Heart Advice for Difficult Times*

🦋 Action Plan 🦋

CHAPTER 3

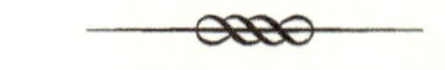

LET'S BE HONEST

"I lied on my Weight Watchers list. I put down that I had three eggs...but they were Cadbury chocolate eggs."
— Caroline Rhea

If you like to watch crime shows or read whodunit books, you know some of the characters don't tell the truth. We kind of expect that. But what about the rest of us when we are asked about weight? Why do we suddenly need an alibi or defense, as though eating chocolate is a crime?

The American Psychiatric Association defines malingering as "the intentional production of false or greatly exaggerated symptoms for the purpose of attaining some identifiable external award."

Use this checklist to see if you fall into the malingering category explaining your behavior and answers you give about weight.

1. You consistently give nearly correct responses to the question "How much do you weigh?" This number is not based on forgetfulness.

2. You are not sick but you quit eating the day before your doctor's visit.

3. The number you give the nurse and the number that is recorded in your chart don't match.

4. When the doctor comes in and mentions your weight, you mention your concern about fluid retention, surprise pregnancy, and other weird things.

5. Your answers cannot be explained by ADHD or side effects of medication for a psychiatric disorder.

It all sounded good at the time.

I hope you can see the humor and the "normalcy" of the checklist. Since this chapter is about honesty, let's talk about resistance to telling the truth about weight. Remember how many diets and plans you've tried? How long did you stick with them? What was the excuse you gave for them not working? What is the real reason?

Was the advertising too enticing, offering instant and unrealistic results? Was it expensive, so *therefore it must be good* kind of thinking? Or "natural" or composed of cabbage or, or, or…?

Or did you really know, in your heart, that you would not be able to do what it said for longer than a week? That's not your fault.

Action Step:

Your action step today is to decide to give this a try. Make a decision. No matter what, you'll try this. You owe it to yourself. I believe in you.

Sit comfortably, close your eyes, and breathe in deeply through your nose and out through your mouth. Become aware of how your body knows how to do this perfectly. Let go.

✹ Action Plan ✹

CHAPTER 4

THE SEDUCTION OF NUMBERS

Your mind produces endless thoughts, feelings, and stories. Mostly, the thoughts are about the past or future, which now only exist as a memory or fantasy. The more attention you give to these stories, the more likely you will suffer. At the very least, you miss out on living in the present moment, which is all we have. Yet, we distract ourselves in a million ways.

Imagine two women sitting on meditation cushions and a bubble over their heads with their thoughts, like you see in cartoons. One woman is thinking, *Woo-hoo! I lost five pounds!* and the other is thinking, *Boo-hoo, I gained five pounds.* What would their teacher say?

"No difference."

Both are lost in judging and thinking. They have lost the joy of living in the present moment.

The number is a number. Period. Can you see the number without creating a story (usually negative) about the number? Don't worry, you won't forget. What I urge you to forget is whether or not it makes you "good."

In mindfulness meditation practice, we are concerned with noticing what's going on right now. Now, that doesn't mean you can no longer think about the past or future, but when you do, you will want to be aware that's what you're doing.

We call the jumping from thought to thought "monkey mind," because when we watch the mind, it seems to leap from one thing to another. The goal is not to stop the monkeys' jumping but to let them jump where they want, while you can observe the thoughts/monkeys without following them.

The easiest thing to do is to come back to your breath.

Action Step:

Counting Breath Meditation (useful for food cravings)

Find a place where you can sit and not be interrupted. Although you can shift around, start with the intention of sitting still. Take a few deep breaths to give the body a signal to relax and then start counting your breaths. Each inhalation and exhalation count as one. Try to develop awareness of the whole breath. When your mind wanders, start again at one for the next breath. This will give you precious minutes to calm your mind and, at the same time, develop mindfulness breathing meditation practice. If you count to ten without your mind wandering, start over. You are developing the willingness to start over again and again.

The practice of counting one's breath can be used as a distraction for food cravings and help you to focus. It will focus your mind and calm the thoughts, and you will learn the lesson of starting again. Like now!

In the beginning, you may only count for a minute or two, but you'll get better with practice. This is a tool you can take with you anywhere, and you can practice this without looking weird.

When you step off the scale, start over.

Zen Koan

Two monks were arguing about the temple flag waving in the wind. One said, "The flag moves." The other said, "The wind moves." They argued back and forth but could not agree. Hui-neng, the Sixth Patriarch, said: "Gentlemen! It is not the flag that moves. It is not the wind that moves. It is your mind that moves." The two monks were struck with awe.

🦋 Action Plan 🦋

CHAPTER 5

YOU'RE A GROWN-UP NOW

Children can only think as children think. We call it egocentric because their thoughts are mostly about them. They also use magical thinking to understand their environment or to play. For children, it is a normal form of delusion. For example, a five-year-old child will say, "I'll be thin and healthy like a fairy princess without doing anything! The fat will just go away tomorrow. I'll wave my magic wand, and I can eat anything I want and not gain weight!"

What is the sound of the adolescent ego? The teenager likes to boast. "I'll never be fat like my father or mother" or "I'll be a runway model or famous entertainer and wear a size four." The teenager's heroic ego has progressed from the childish magical thinking but still leaves out harsh realities of life. Then again, the adolescent thinking style does bring hope, and we all need hope. How would it be if someone told us at the beginning of our weight loss journey, "Look, this is hard work. It is likely you are not happy in all areas of your life, and losing weight is a big task that will take energy, devotion, and commitment." Without hope, it could feel scary or as boring as "Let's all do taxes."

So, how do you face, realistically, your need to lose weight and drop your magical thinking and keep your heroic hopes and proceed?

You can do it now.

Everyone reading this book has hope and knowledge. Your hope is based on what you imagine yourself to be, hope to be. Knowledge is the value of what you've learned about yourself and your approach to weight.

Wisdom, from Socrates' approach, is humbling. It is the knowing that we do not know. Wisdom frees us from the "this or that" thinking. We do not have to be "right." Through hope and knowledge, we can become wise. Wisdom points us in the right direction.

Action Step:

What else do you need to know? What else do you need to do? Write your answers in a journal. Commit to one action step. Look at your resistance to change. What are you afraid of becoming? Doing? This is where the suffering lies, in resistance to having what you want.

The Buddha

"We practice meditation in order to see ourselves as we truly are and life as it truly is. When we are suffering, we can look inside to find the cause—always some form of clinging. By noticing how quickly we attach to new ideas and perspectives, we can begin to unlearn the habit. One trick is to watch for moments when we feel the need to defend ourselves or our point of view. Defensiveness is always a red flag; it shows that we have once again become stuck in a point of view. We are pretending to be solid, and we want everyone else to go along with it. With a little honesty and effort, we can determine where we are stuck and then choose to let go. Gradually we become more flexible, finding it easier to let go of our perspectives. We take this 'me' less seriously, appreciating instead our dynamic and unfixed true nature.

With practice, we begin to see the world from the perspective of BIG MIND, which can see all perspectives but clings to none. We learn that it is possible to return to the view of BIG MIND whenever we've become stuck. It's easiest to assume that we're stuck somewhere; we only have to figure out where and then let go. Liberation from the self is living each day without a place to stand or ideas about who we are. That's when we can dance with life."

—Genpo Roshi, *The Path of the Human Being*

🦋 Action Plan 🦋

CHAPTER 6

BREAKING UP

Certain conditions must exist for a rainbow to appear. Can you think of your body in the same way? What condition had to exist for a pound to appear?

We see a rainbow in its totality, not only pink or red or blue color. Can you expand that idea to your body? You are not the weight of an arm, a belly, or a foot. A body is not fragmented except in our perception. Each pound appears with all other pounds.

That said, the pounds leave one by one. If you fear losing weight, you might clutch at them like a fearful child, feeling abandoned. If the pounds don't leave fast enough, by our standards, you may feel hopeless, yearning for things to be different. No peace of mind either way.

It could be helpful for you to examine how you have reacted to breakups in personal relationships. Unless you can understand the pattern, reasons, problems, you tend to look for another person and find one similar to the one you just had. We don't want this to happen in the breakup with your weight. Keeping extra pounds is similar to staying in a relationship that's not healthy for you.

Some people never break up.

Look at your relationship with food and habits. Look at the habits, beliefs, and foods that maintain your weight. Love yourself. Loving yourself will give you the strength to leave a bad relationship, change your life, and enjoy the romance of loving yourself, totally.

Love Your Rainbow!

Action Step:

Wake up full, not of food, but of yourself. Rediscover yourself every day and then forget yourself. You will not be forgotten.

Chuang-Tsu

The purpose of a fish trap is to catch fish, and when the fish are caught, the trap is forgotten. The purpose of a rabbit snare is to catch rabbits. When the rabbits are caught, the snare is forgotten. The purpose of words is to convey ideas. When the ideas are grasped, the words are forgotten. Where can I find a man who has forgotten words? He is the one I would like to talk to.

🦋 Action Plan 🦋

CHAPTER 7

UNDERSTANDING THE COST OF LOSS

While you say you want to lose weight, can you acknowledge that change (losing weight) involves loss of something else? This change will have an effect on loved ones, friends, coworkers, and acquaintances. Some of them may even miss the "old you" and miss your old body and personality characteristics. They may think you are sick. They may feel envy and be inspired to take care of their own health now.

Give yourself time. This is nothing new as the real you has always lived in your mind. However, it may be time to believe "you" have arrived. Let go of old habits and give yourself time to embrace the new habits, feelings, and ways of living on your terms.

As you lose weight, you will gain some things too. You will gain health, confidence, and pleasure in the forgotten (aromas, nature). And how about some new clothes?

You must gain something or else you would not keep putting in so much effort, money, and time in the hope of—what? It is likely not a number on the scale. It is likely things unseen but known to you.

Action Step:

Meditate on the intention to reduce anxiety about your body change. When thoughts arise about the future, let them go by like a cloud in the sky and come back to the breath. If the mind wanders a thousand times, gently bring it back a thousand times.

Chogyam Trungpa Rinpoche, From "Ground," in *Glimpses of Shunyata*
Follow the truth of the way.
Reflect on it. Make it your own.
Live it.
It will always sustain you.
Do not turn away what is given you, nor reach out for what is given to others,
Lest you disturb your quietness.

❧ Action Plan ❧

CHAPTER 8

WRITING YOUR THANK-YOU NOTE

What does the sound of one pound dropping sound like at family dinners or whenever dining out with friends? It sounds like finding joy in things and people other than food. The environment is more than the food. There is conversation and laughter to enjoy. Even the crying babies knit the experience of togetherness that satisfies more than the taste of food. Next time, imagine these things are on the menu too.

Action 1: Write a thank-you note to your overweight "Fat Self" for being your friend and enemy. It may be that you'll miss all the excuses that Fat Self gave you to stay home, not dress up, avoid people and activities. Leave out blame, anger, and shame. Be polite.

Action 2: Write a Dear John letter to Fat. Break up. Apologize that you can't take Fat Self to any more parties, friends' houses, or have him/her hang around in your kitchen. Write until you feel you've broken up for good.

Action 3: Make a list of places to send your Fat clothes.

❦ Action Plan ❦

CHAPTER 9

WHERE DO YOU FIT?

Have you noticed how many institutions supporting diet and weight loss aids are part of our social fabric? You can readily bring to mind commercial ads, books, products, support groups, magazines, exercise machines, spas and health clubs that cater to the problem of overweight people. All promise results. Some brands/businesses claim they help, but the fact that they are still in business tells us most people fail or need more and more of the product to lose weight.

Currently, there is a new push growing in our society toward prevention of obesity. There are campaigns urging people to develop and maintain fitness and health. The shift may sound subtle, but it is huge. People who are not overweight or do not have health problems are now bombarded with the same ads, books, magazines, etc. to maintain what they already have.

Where do you fit? Ads and fads are cyclical, but you are not. Today is the day to rise above extremes and negative messages and end the craving for a "perfect" size. Read that again.

Today is the day to form your own ideas about your optimistic but realistic goals for your body and mental state. You can do this without any outside advice. Dwell with these thoughts today and notice how free you can feel when you trust your own intuition and knowledge. You know what to do and how to do it. Begin.

Steppingstone: Guided Meditation

The stones are laid out to cross the river to the other side. You may be able to skip some, step over others; you slip off, feel stuck, but you know all you have to do is pick your next steppingstone and find your footing. There. Breathe.

Action Step:

Record your goals in a journal. Do you want to eat six small meals a day? Write that down. Do you want to maintain your weight? Weigh daily and record your numbers. Be brave and start a food diary. Write down what you eat and how you feel during the day. You will not do this forever, but writing now gets the momentum going, and you'll feel more like adding to your journal entries if you commit to staying with it for a couple of weeks. After that, the spirit will move you or you'll have developed a good habit. The diary is not to serve as a shame and guilt log; it is a nonjudgmental account of events in your life—and it matters.

> **Everything**
> **just as it is,**
> **as it is,**
> **as is.**
> **Flowers in bloom.**
> **Nothing to add.**
> —Robert Aitken Roshi, "*As It Is*"

🦋 Action Plan 🦋

CHAPTER 10

RETHINKING FOOD AND FEELINGS: WHAT ARE YOU REALLY EATING?

"I am not overweight. I am in the
process of becoming thin."

—Former client

Thoughts change the chemistry of your body. Thoughts that evoke feelings of anger release stress hormones. They ripple across your body, leaving it agitated and tense. There is a sense of holding on to all you have, including weight. Sad thoughts or negative thoughts elicit their own messages from the body. It's everyone's problem. But it is a solvable problem.

What is the problem? We say food is the problem. Food is not the problem. We say people are the problem, but they are not the problem. What is the problem? Being overweight? Being overweight is not the problem. What is the problem? The problem is the feelings and thoughts about food, your body, and being overweight.

What do you believe about food? Is it scarce? Harmful? Good or addictive? How do you feel about food being scarce? Do you feel mad, good, pleased, or trapped? Is it true that you have to let yourself feel scared around certain foods? Is food an enemy to be conquered? No.

Is your body an enemy? No. Your body is you and the result of your choices. Your body has changed as a result of your choices, and it can and will change more as a result of your choices. It's up to you. Taste hope.

Today, let go again. Some people find that doing something physical helps to "work it out." A gentler release is yoga, meditation, or guided imagery techniques.

Anger and sadness weigh heavy on your heart. What is the sound of feelings leaving? A sigh of relief.

Action Steps:

Write down situations, events, or people that evoke a feeling (such as anger, resentment, hurt, shame, sadness, etc.). If you are angry at yourself, put yourself first on the list. Add all the memories that pop up when you stay with this question.

Now, tear the list up slowly, and feel with every rip all the feelings dissolving. Let it go. Let it go. Shake your hands as though you are trying to dry them without a towel.

In your meditation practice today, and while you are going about daily life, reflect on the words "let go." It might help to open your hands or lift them when you are able to do this as a way to release any tension. Please treat yourself and your body kindly and well.

You are in charge and you have hope.

🦋 Action Plan 🦋

CHAPTER 11

ENVY AND HUNGER

Envy can be a good thing. Envy is recognizing that something another person has would be good for you too. For example, I see a woman with a purple dress, and I think it looks lovely on her. I do not want her purple dress, but I think one like hers would look good on me. I have no desire to take her purple dress away from her.

Envy has a feeling tone of yearning or hunger for something. We hunger after what the other person has, such as a thin, healthy body and purple dresses.

Envy affects the envier. Unless we understand the positive side of envy, we can feel persecuted by seemingly always seeing thin people and other things that catch our attention. Advertisements have to create envy to get us to buy their product. It can feel overwhelming.

So where do you go when you feel you are being dragged under? Can you find a way out to connect to satisfying experiences in yourself rather than spend time imagining them in others?

There is a paradox of dreading having what one desires, for then one becomes the envied. As long as the thinness is outside the person, the indulgence of envy can continue.

Follow the envy if it is what you have perceived as good. Although you see it outside yourself, it is what you intuitively know is either in you as well or it is something you desire.

Envy can use up our lives. It keeps our sense of self, our egos captive. We must claim this part of our personalities to escape the energy of it. Air it in the light of day. Bring it to consciousness.

Action Step:

Practice gratitude. Cultivate a practice of gratefulness for help, seeing success in others to give us inspiration. Let yourself have new experiences.

Let each bite of food taste like the first bite. Realize the mystery of food and be grateful for its existence. Enjoy the colors of food, the smells, and the textures. Be grateful for the nutrients that feed us.

🦋 Action Plan 🦋

CHAPTER 12

THE LANDSCAPE OF OUR LIVES AND FOOD

We are born into landscapes, and the landscapes inform us. Think about your childhood landscape. What did you see when you looked out the window? What sounds did you hear?

Where did everyone work? If you lived on farmland, chances are no one around was a commercial fisherman, which meant you ate more beef than fish. If you lived near the sea, you probably ate more fish than potatoes.

Not only does the landscape shape what becomes familiar, but it also shapes our food choices and what tastes like "home cooking." Was it beef, fish, chicken, peaches, or pecans? Does this explain why I always choose fried okra on any menu? Probably.

What are the foods of your landscape? What smells filled the kitchen?

But isn't vacation great? Isn't it fun to taste foods from other cultures and countries? What started as "the front yard" has turned into the yards of the world. We're all alike in cultivating tastes of our home.

Action Step:

Write your answers in your journal. Reflect on what you wrote. Finally, look for the thread of desire when you reach for _______________________ to satisfy a hunger.

Did you eat this to distract yourself?

Who gave it to you as a child?

Who enjoyed cooking, serving, eating these foods? How are your feelings connected to these people, these times, this place?

Conversely, who did not enjoy cooking and how did this impact you?

Do you think eating childhood foods is a way you connect to the people who cooked for you?

Is there another way you can connect other than food?

Perhaps an object that is a metaphor for the feeling of home-cooked meals or feeling cared for by someone. A special glass? A spice? A picture? You'll come up with the perfect object that means something to you.

After doing this reflective exercise, what did you learn about yourself?

✖ Action Plan ✖

CHAPTER 13

REMEMBERING "I AM THAT"

Have you ever said, "That's not like me," as though there is only one way to be you? We tend to say, "She's just like me" as a way of saying we like a person based on a narrow perception of her (or him). But how does weight change your choices of finding someone "just like me," and how might you sabotage your weight loss when you can't find or accept someone different as "just like me"?

Philosophers and psychologists give us a reason for this behavior. We meet ourselves in the other. However, when you are overweight, you give up that experience of "I am that" or "I'm like her" with people who have a physique you wish to have. Even if you remember having a similar physique, you experience "I am not that; I am not like her." But you are.

You must remember when you meet others of normal weight that "I am that too" and enjoy the engagement of your alter ego. This shift allows your alter ego to remember or get used to the idea of "she's just like me when I'm thinner." And, not to show bias, when you meet someone heavier, because "she's just like me if I were heavier."

Action Step:

For an exercise: look at strangers with the intentional thought of *I am that too*. Notice the chatter in the mind. Afterward, take some time to do calming meditation by sitting with the breath. Not thinking about past or future but gently calming the mind with intentional single-point concentration on the breath.

🦋 Action Plan 🦋

CHAPTER 14

IMPERMANENCE

There was a time when you were not this weight. You remember it. You may long for it and even suffer for it.

Impermanence.

Let that word linger in front of your mind. The weight you are today will not be the weight you will be for all your life. Don't argue. Even throughout the day your weight goes up and down. It is part of our human existence, indeed, our nature to change.

Every action has a consequence. If you have a pebble in your shoe and you put more weight on the other foot to avoid pain, there will be a consequence. The lesson is to accept what is there and remove the pebble today. Take one small step in creating an action that has a favorable consequence. One has already come to mind.

Action Step:

Let's go shopping! Find a catalog or website with clothes you like. Pick out an outfit to symbolize "you" at your desired weight. Now pick out another one that symbolizes your style. Now pick out an outfit that is outrageous, but, if you had __________, you would feel special. It's okay if you purchase it, or you can own it in your imagination. Let that outfit hang in your closet; see yourself wearing it. After all, life is about impermanence. What is meaningful and beautiful to you today may not be tomorrow, but who cares? Embrace impermanence.

🦋 Action Plan 🦋

CHAPTER 15

SOLVE YOUR WEIGHT RIDDLE AT ANY AGE

Did someone tell you that you can't lose weight when you get "older"? And what age is that, anyway? If you're tempted to use age as an excuse for keeping your same weight…um, nope, we're not going to go there. Even if you argue that you just want it to end, it's not fair, or any other cliché you like, we do have to talk about it.

Even though aging is something that we all do, our society treats it as a disease. It is not. Today, we'll sort through your emotions about aging and weight. It is possible to have peace of mind and face your feelings.

Yes, I know. You never planned to be overweight at this age. It's not "you."

Answer this question: do you know what you need to do about losing weight? Really think about your answer. Push away your resentments and resistance, and quit telling yourself you'll be "all right." No, you won't be all right. You've got to have the heart to make these changes for your life.

Tell the truth. Have realistic expectations. Take on something you can do without beating yourself up. Change what you can. And it's okay if you don't quite know all the answers. We are all uncertain. No one has all the answers.

Sometimes we go through the stages one goes through with loss when we lose weight. In the first stage you feel shock and say things that put off coming face-to-face with the task of losing weight. "Why do I have to do it now?" "Well, I walk all day." Then comes the second stage of anger and depression. Once you begin to acknowledge the impact of overeating on your health and well-being, you will likely feel angry and depressed. Mood swings, though painful, are good teachers. Feel what you are feeling, feel sad, don't bottle up your feelings, and be gentle but firm.

Do something different and constructive to acknowledge your feelings. Sing loudly, journal your thoughts, draw with crayons, meditate daily. Stage four is acceptance and understanding. Acceptance means being at peace with losing weight and living well. Understanding this fact honors our humanness. Many people attach themselves to the idea of thinner and younger. You won't get younger. You will get thinner and healthier—and older. Sorry if that's a bit of joy mixed with sorrow for you. Losing weight does not have to be a terrible time! Let go of the "if onlys."

Action Step:

Write a letter to your body and list all your regrets. Here is an example:

> Dear Body,
>
> I regret that I stuffed you for years. I regret never giving you enough sleep. I regret not taking you for enough walks. You would have enjoyed that. I regret... Fill in the blank.

The final part of this exercise is to imagine your body forgiving you. Close your eyes and imagine yourself/body saying what you most need to hear right now. Do it several times a day.

Each time you do this, open your hands and shake them, letting the energy or thoughts release. Let go.

Action Plan

CHAPTER 16

NONVIOLENT ANSWERS

Weight loss does not have to be violent or punitive. Give up forcing false food and pills down your throat.

Release any pressures you feel to please, change, or meet someone's image of you.

Stop torturing your body and mind. Let peace of mind return.

Just for today, give up planning, predicting, and most of all, desiring. Unmet expectations bring suffering.

Clear a space for happiness. Pick flowers from your yard and place them in your line of sight. Even a weed is beautiful.

Weight loss comes at its own time. We can predict, plan, and desire, but that brings suffering from unmet expectations and false happiness when it meets expectations. It disturbs peace of mind.

Action Step:

For today, practice nonviolent care of your body. Continue caring for your food, environment, and body. Have a curious mind about your body weight. Get close to the feelings living in your body. Be gentle in your evaluations.

❧ Action Plan ❧

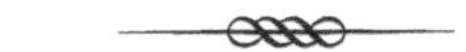

CHAPTER 17

WHY WE ASSUME FAT PEOPLE ARE HAPPY

It is because people wear a mask much like a clown's mask. The real person is behind the mask, living on the other side, looking out. You see, a fat person does not want to claim the identity of a fat person, does not want that to be who they are. So, they are trapped into playing a role. It is an act.

Well, "So what?" you ask. It is exhausting. Guess what we do when we are tired and exhausted? We eat, drink, numb out. Guess what we do when we leave the stage and go to our own home? We eat, drink, numb out. Alone and feeling unloved and unlovable.

What happens when the office or family clown goes away? Do they say hurrah? No, they want the fat, funny clown there to amuse them, to reflect their own emotions and life, but not for the clown to have one of her own.

There's always an extra mask around in case someone puts on a few pounds. They'll hear: "See, I told you so... After forty you'll be fat like the rest of the family. Here's your mask. Be happy."

What is the sound of one pound dropping? It is the sound of listening, seeing, and changing. It is the sound of the fairy-tale book closing gently on this part of life. It is the sound of sitting with our loneliness, letting new visions emerge into our dreams, consciousness, lives.

Action Step:

You can be happy at any weight, size, age, race, gender, nationality. You are not defined by others.

Define yourself. What makes you happy? What parts of yourself do you hide from others to please them, to get them to like you?

Take one small step today being your authentic self. Don't smile if you don't feel it. Don't eat it if you don't like it.

🦋 Action Plan 🦋

CHAPTER 18

NONVIOLENT WEIGHT LOSS

If you were to starve someone (like yourself) or force-feed them false food and pills, it would be considered violent torture. Yet, people do it to themselves all the time by twisting themselves into an image of another, agreeing to eat what is prescribed or mailed to them in the hope that pain will have a payoff.

Even with negative feedback from these attempts, do you still yearn for the magic pill or injection that will change your body? If your body could speak, what would it say about that?

What is the sound of someone in agony? Feelings have sounds. The moans of pain, the sighs of depression, the arrrggh! of frustration are clues to something deeper than the sound.

Feelings have inner, quiet sounds too. The ones we hold in but listen to. Messages and repeating phrases about who you are, what you do, and where you failed are all there. No wonder you will do almost anything or eat anything to distract and comfort yourself. If only that helped…but you know from experience that it intensifies the pain and the agony. And the inner sound of guilt, blame, anger, shame, and humiliation begin their chorus: "You failed, you cheated on your diet, stole a doughnut, and you're stupid." You may have a different verse, but it all amounts to making you feel bad and alone.

There are other ways. There are other verses to sing. Just for today, give up planning, predicting, and most of all, dieting. Release any pressures you feel to please, change, or meet someone's image of you. Stop torturing yourself. Have your own protest sit-in!

Let peace of mind return. Clear a space for happiness. Weight loss comes in its own time. We can predict, plan, and desire, but that brings suffering from unmet expectations and false happiness when it meets expectations. It disturbs your peace of mind.

Action Step:

For today, practice nonviolent care of your body. Continue caring for your food, environment, and body. Have a curious mind about your weight. Get close to the feelings about your weight and health. Be gentle in your evaluations. It's simply a result of past choices.

Whose expectations are you trying to meet? Write about that in your journal. Acknowledge that the past is the past.

And forgiveness is welcomed here.

🦋 Action Plan 🦋

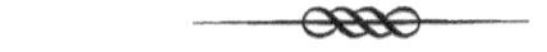

CHAPTER 19

BENEFITS FROM MEDITATION PRACTICE

Meditation is a spiritual and personal practice that has existed for eons in all parts of the world. Research shows that consistent meditation practice can restore mental capacity and function, alleviate various health conditions, and improve memory. People intuited this long before scientists proved it, but if you need any convincing that this may be good for you, the scientific research is there for you to see.

Here are some of the benefits gleaned from the research:

Stress Management

Meditation practice helps manage stress because it slows down your breathing and teaches you to focus your attention by following your breath and/or thoughts. Some people recite a mantra, prayer, or affirmation or count breaths in and out. Any of these will help you solve problems in new ways.

Improves Cognitive Function

Practicing meditation has been shown to alter the structure and function of the brain, which is what allows us to learn and improve memory.

Wellness

Meditation has been shown to give relief for people with insomnia, anxiety, depression, high blood pressure, and more. Stopping intrusive thoughts will result in better state of mind and overall health.

Addiction

Meditation-based therapy helps people addicted to foods, drugs, or alcohol. Mindfulness meditation shows us that feelings do not have to determine behavior. Being aware of how cravings come and go can enhance the ability to resist them.

Spirit

Meditation can be a spiritual practice. Feeling closer to Spirit, God, Universe, or Nature offers a sense of belonging, care, and peace.

For what you will get from investing a small amount of time developing a meditation practice, I think that's a pretty good bargain.

🦋 Action Plan 🦋

C H A P T E R   2 0

BON VOYAGE!
SEND YOUR CRAVINGS AWAY

Let's have a party!

Cravings are like uninvited guests at your party. They show up when you are worried, sad, happy, or excited. In other words, they are attached to your emotions. They are old friends, often formed in childhood when you discovered they comforted you. Like old friends, you have your favorites. Salty ones? Sweets? Alcohol? They have served you well, but you are ready to send them on a well-deserved vacation. All aboard!

Make a list of their names. Ice cream, Cookies, Candy, etc. You'll hear from them from time to time, but you won't invite them to stay at your house or allow them to show up uninvited.

Action Step:

In your journal, write your old friends a thank-you note. Acknowledge their role in your life and how they have helped, and yet sabotaged, your health. Tell them you are taking a break from their company and wish them well.

Next, make a list of all the things you can do instead of indulging in cravings for your "old friends." Include doing things for others, such as taking someone a small bouquet of flowers for their house/office.

Celebrate freedom.

Action Step:

Give yourself the gift of time to practice meditation.

❀ Action Plan ❀

CHAPTER 21

SMALL STEPS COUNT

Baby steps. Progress, not perfection. You've heard it before because it is true. Please don't dismiss them as clichés but rather adopt them as affirmations.

Think about how much happiness is expressed when a baby takes a first step. Parents rejoice! They encourage the baby to do it again. They call people and take pictures of the baby walking. It is a developmental milestone. A Big Deal.

Your baby steps are just as important. Years of not trusting yourself to celebrate a good day or feeling depressed if you don't meet a goal have conditioned you to not trust your instincts to celebrate your own progress. No more.

Everything counts. If you've cleaned out the sugar bowl and substituted sugar with Stevia or another product, you won't have to make a decision every time you add sugar to something. Easy peasy. Your turn.

Action Step:

Record your baby steps in your journal. It could be that you stretched your body or ate a piece of fruit for a healthy snack. Maybe you allowed yourself to sleep or rest, gave yourself a facial, or noticed you had the freedom to do nothing, which is also "something."

In formal Zen meditation practice, people sit facing a wall. How long do you think it takes for the lesson to be learned that the wall is a wall, and no matter how much you wish it was different, it remains true to being a wall. Notice how your mind may want things to be different, easier, quicker. Let your life today be like the wall. It is what it is. When will you be satisfied?

🦋 Action Plan 🦋

CHAPTER 22

LOVE IS IN YOUR MIND

Like Tina Turner's song, "What's Love Got To Do With It?" you may be wondering what love has to do with getting healthier, losing weight, or any other personal change you want to make. It makes a huge difference. For example, imagine a stranger giving you a bouquet of flowers. Nice, but unless the stranger really grabs your attention, the gesture will soon be forgotten. You do not fall in love with the stranger, right? Play along with me here. Imagine you go on a fancy dinner date with fine dining, music, flowers with someone who does not grab your attention in the least. You may enjoy the meal, but you are not in love with the dinner date. Because love lives in your mind. It matters what you think about what/who you see.

That's why it is important to love the person in the mirror. You. Love will not come from a salad or a smoothie. Those are nice but they miss the mark when it comes to a feeling of love. Why is it so many people settle for this? We're judgmental. We hold beliefs about ourselves that are self-defeating, or have unrealistic versions of "what I should look like" to be lovable.

Most people could use a little coaching on building a loving relationship with themselves. You wouldn't call other people bad

65

names if you wanted to get to know them better, would you? You might even offer compliments to them when they least expect it to get the relationship moving in the right direction, wouldn't you?

Action Step:

What can you do today—just one thing—that elevates the person in the mirror to an equal status worthy of your respect, love, and care. I promise you'll enjoy hanging out together.

🦋 Action Plan 🦋

CHAPTER 23

HOW TO USE MANTRAS AND QUOTES

A mantra can be a phrase you've heard all your life as well as an intentionally created one.

OM is a mantra. It is pronounced o-ah-mum. It is a mantra chanted by Buddhists and non-Buddhists alike. Try it out while meditating. Pay attention to how it vibrates in your mouth and down your throat and chest wall. It feels similar to humming, which is a good way to release stress.

"Amen" is another word used as a mantra. In prayer, in agreements, we say Amen, Amen.

Quotes can become a supportive reminder throughout the day. They move you. They say something true in a few words. You can choose them. Collect them like shells you find on a deserted beach seemingly washed up for your eyes only.

Action Step:

Go on a treasure hunt today and begin to collect lines of lyrics, poems, and full quotes that sing to your soul, such as this line from

Mary Oliver's poem, "What will you do with your one and only precious life?"

Write them, keep them, choose one to memorize and then another, until you have them in your soul to travel the day with you.

✠ Action Plan ✠

CHAPTER 24

HOW LONG DOES IT TAKE

How long does it take you to notice the number on the scale and judge yourself? How long does it take you to become aware of your thoughts and feelings about your body? How long does it take to create a meaning for the number you see on the scale? It can happen in the blink of an eye, can't it?

This is an obsessive pattern: see, judge, shame. The good news is that you can be released from this obsessive pattern by understanding the ongoing seesaw between shame and acceptance. No matter which way the mind goes, there is never enough shame. There is never enough acceptance. Until you change the pattern. Get off the seesaw.

Can you let go of the need to clean your plate? Probably, until the next time. Can you let go of spending your precious life moments feeling discouraged or on top of the world, till the next time?

In this one moment of your life, how do you wish to spend it? And the next moment?

Action Step:

Mindfulness Practice. Mindfulness practice is an exercise that has scientific validity to change your life, and even your brain. It is an exercise just like any physical exercise. It takes willingness to notice. It is not about relaxation or even harmony and peace. Some of life just isn't that way. What will happen as you practice just five minutes a day for three days a week is that you will become curious about your thoughts and feelings, noticing and coming back to your breath. What will your mind think about that? You'll be surprised. Once you notice your thoughts nonjudgmentally, you will generalize this in your waking life. So, here is a short version of this action step.

1. Sit with your feet on the floor, straight, like a ribbon is attached to your head and the ceiling, gently holding your head still with your eyes straight ahead, closed if you wish.

2. Notice that you are breathing! Focus on how the air comes in and out of your nostrils; follow your breath inside and exhale, sensing you are releasing into the room. Continue. When you notice a thought, come back to the breath. Some people imagine a fishing pole gently reeling your attention back to the breath. Others visualize a cloud with thoughts, with the wind blowing it away. Some people like a more kinesthetic approach by making a hand gesture, centering the hands over the heart... Play around with what works for you. The point is always the same: bring your attention back to the breath, without judgment, over and over again.

At the end of five minutes, write about your experience today. Was there something that came up that surprised you? Annoyed you? Was it ho-hum? There is no right or wrong, remember—no judgments, just acceptance.

Action Plan

CHAPTER 25

LETTING GO OF THE WEIGHT OF YOUR PAST

You grew up hearing family stories. They impact you. I'm asking you now to assume a curious attitude and use this exercise to learn more about yourself. To begin, gather small objects, such as pebbles, pennies, buttons, or dry beans. You will use these to designate what histories have shaped your family and you.

Take a large sheet of paper and begin drawing your family tree. Use squares for men and circles for women, or you can draw stick figures. Go back three generations or as much as you can remember. You'll want your immediate family, your cousins, your grandparents, your great-grandparents, and any other aunts and uncles you know or have heard about. You can use lines to connect people, broken lines to indicate divorce or estranged people. You can write a letter "D" to indicate deceased, and if you know the cause of their death, write that in too.

Now, ask yourself, Which relatives were riddled with grief or distress? Place your small object over their name or close by. You may see that there are few people in your family who did not suffer grief.

Second question: Which relatives met with a tragic fate, such as accidental or homicidal death or early illness? Again, place a pebble near their name.

Third question: Did any children die? Place a pebble by their name.

Fourth question: Was anyone in the family disowned or considered themselves the black sheep?

Fifth question: Did anyone in the family go to war?

Sixth question: Did anyone in the family go to jail?

Seventh question: Did anyone in the family emigrate under threat?

Eighth question: Did anyone become, at times, violent? Or suffer from someone's violence?

Ninth question: Did anyone in the family tree experience poverty at some time in their lives?

Tenth question: Did anyone suffer from political oppression?

Eleventh question: Did anyone in the family suffer from addiction (drugs, alcohol, food, gambling, gaming, work)?

Twelfth question: Did anyone in the family suffer from abuse (physical, emotional, or sexual)?

Thirteenth question: Was anyone in the family obese or anorexic?

Step back and look at the big picture. Each person affects other people in the family, and we may wind up carrying their shame or issues as our own as a way to "honor" them.

Write in your journal or say out loud how you are ending this family story and will no longer _____ (overeat, starve, drink, etc.) as you move on with your life as a healthy and independent family member.

Use the journal to write more about your feelings. For instance, in my case, my father's brother was killed in an accident when he was twelve years old. My father was fourteen at the time. His mother told him she wished it had been him and more terrible things, which, in turn, changed him and how he related to my own mother once she became "mother" to me.

At the end of this exercise, only keep the pebbles that are yours. You can declare the family pebbles as not yours and that you will no longer feel that they are. Every life has tragedies. The things that happened to your family did not happen to you. Underline that sentence.

Choose.

Action Plan

www.ingramcontent.com/pod-product-compliance
Lightning Source LLC
Chambersburg PA
CBHW022057150726
47990CB00003B/1128